THE ULTIMATE DASH DIET COOKBOOK

WITH 50 SIMPLE BUT DELICIOUS RECIPES TO HELP LOWER YOUR BLOOD PRESSURE AND IMPROVE YOUR HEART HEALTH

Table of Contents

Introduction

What Is The Dash Diet?

When the DASH study and the DASH sodium study were carried out more than two decades ago, it wasn't done to come up with a diet to promote weight loss. The researchers involved wanted to help hypertensive patients with a diet that also acted as an effective medicine. That being the case, weight reduction is presently the most famous aspect of this particular eating plan.

Companies and blogs who sell DASH inspired products often like to focus on the fact this diet will help you shed the extra pounds you've been battling to lose.

Not only will you be able to lose the unwanted pounds but, if you follow the diet with discipline, you will do so much faster than imagined.

And it shouldn't surprise you that the DASH diet can accomplish this. DASH is both a diet and a lifestyle. As such, you not only have to be mindful of what goes into your mouth. You are also expected to control how you conduct yourself.

DASH: The Diet

Three excellent factors make this eating plan great for those who want to look slimmer. Let's consider each of them.

Healthy fats

The first is that you are expected only to consume healthy fats. Good fats, as they are so often called.

You mustn't generalize and think all fats are bad for you. Even though it is a wide-spread belief that all fats will make it so you can no longer see your feet and endows you with a second chin, this isn't a fact.

The fats you should stay away from are trans-fat and saturated fat. All those scary things they have accused every type of fat of causing, trans and saturated fat are the actual culprits. Think about it: obesity, an increased risk of suffering hypertension and cancer, clogged arteries, and other kinds of heart disease. It's as a result of consuming those bad fats.

This doesn't mean that throwing caution to the wind and eating without any discipline doesn't play a role in causing these health conditions. But you greatly increase your risk by eating such artificial fats.

On the other hand, good fats are exactly what your body needs. These good or healthy fats include omega-3s and unsaturated fats. You know those times when you feel so tired, you can barely lift your hand as you lie in bed? Or the mornings you just get pissed at things that wouldn't matter to you on a good day? Your body very well may have been screaming for good fats.

Their many benefits including keeping your mind as sharp as a katana blade, giving you control over which way your mood should swing, helping you stay active all day, and promoting weight loss.

You read that right. Consuming unsaturated fats will help you lose those calories faster and healthier than if you try to do without them. Just as people get fats wrong, they also do the same with cholesterol. It has been so vilified at this point, that the mere mention of its name probably gives you heartburn. In reality, your entire body system would be thrown into chaos without cholesterol. The problem is when you consume too much of it. In life, if anything exceeds the bounds of moderation, then it is very likely dangerous. Your body also follows the same rule. Too little cholesterol and you might need to visit the doctor. Moderate cholesterol and your body will thank you for it. Too much cholesterol and you are making goo-goo eyes at the Grim Reaper.

To control your cholesterol levels, you should watch the fats you consume. Sticking with only healthy fats is a good way to make sure your cholesterol level stays moderate. And choosing the DASH diet is the overall best way to maintain a healthy intake of good fats.

High-fiber

Fiber is such an amazing nutrient; surprisingly, we don't eat it as often as we should. Most of the DASH diet foods are rich in both soluble and insoluble fibers, which is perfect for anyone dealing with digestive issues. Grains, fruits, vegetables, and legumes are some of the places where fiber is found in high quantities. If your grandma, or anyone else in your family, offered you some vegetables as a home remedy for constipation, then you've experienced one of the many benefits of consuming fiber. Did you know that the body can neither break down nor absorb fiber? It is unlike every other nutrient you take into your body. For example, fats are broken down into fatty acids and glycerol, and carbohydrates are broken down into glucose. Fibers just pass through your entire digestive system relatively unchanged. Again, fibers can be soluble or insoluble. This means they either dissolve in water or not. Soluble fibers, found in oats, apples, carrots, etc. are good for reducing cholesterol and glucose levels in the blood. Insoluble fibers, on the other hand, are helpful to individuals who are dealing with constipation. It also promotes stool bulk. You will find insoluble fibers in food sources like cauliflower and potatoes. While fibers absorb the water in your stool (Not something you want to read about? It'll be over soon) and make them bulky instead of loose, they also make them soft. As a result, your risk of getting hemorrhoids is reduced. Also, as common as diverticular disease is, you can avoid getting it. You may think it's no big deal, but you could suffer abdominal pain if those small pouches in your intestinal walls become inflamed.

Suppose that isn't incentive enough for you to start chowing down on some fruits, veggies, and legumes. In that case, you should know that a high-fiber diet helps lower your risk of colorectal cancer. Some scientists even believe that dietary fiber may be useful to prevent many colon diseases (Mayo Clinic, 2018). There is ongoing research to prove this. The deal-breaker for you could be this: switching to a high-fiber diet will prevent your blood sugar from spiking. As a result, and because your digestion has now been improved, fat will not be stored in your belly.

Are you familiar with DASH Diet? Do you want to know more about Instant Pot cooking? Do you want to have over 180 easy, healthy and delicious DASH Diet recipes to lose weight and better your life? This book will give you answers! This is where Dash Diet (Dietary Approach to Stop Hypertension) is unique. Unlike other diets, the core objective of a Dash Diet is not to trim you down, but rather to help you lower your blood pressure and prevents hypertension and other cardiovascular diseases.

What is even more interesting is the fact that positive results can be experienced just after two weeks after starting the diet! Unlike other diets, you won't have to sacrifice your favorite foods in order to follow it! While a Dash Diet primarily focuses on increasing the intake of fruits, vegetables, low fat dairy items and a good amount of grains. It doesn't necessarily force you to become a complete vegetarian as red meats and fish are acceptable, albeit in small quantities.

The key thing to remember with a Dash Diet is to strike the perfect balance where your maximum sodium intake is limited to 1500mg per day. To put that into perspective, a typical American diet consists of more than 3,400 mg per day!

Recipes

Breakfast

1 Chickpeas Salad

Preparation time: 10 minutes

Cooking time: 0 minutes

Servings: 4

Ingredients:

1 tablespoon parsley, chopped

1 tablespoon mint, chopped

1 tablespoon chives, chopped

2 ounces radishes, chopped

2 beets, peeled and grated

1 apple, cored, peeled and cubed

1 teaspoon cumin, ground

2 ounces quinoa, cooked

3 tablespoons olive oil

7 ounces canned chickpeas, no-salt-added, drained and rinsed

7 ounces canned green chilies, chopped

Juice of 2 lemons

Directions:

In a bowl, combine the parsley with the mint, chives, radishes, beets, apple, cumin, quinoa, oil, chickpeas, chilies and lemon juice, toss well, divide into small bowls and serve for breakfast.

Enjoy!

Nutrition: calories 251, fat 8, fiber 8, carbs 14, protein 14

2 Delicious Blueberry Breakfast Salad

Preparation time: 10 minutes

Cooking time: 0 minutes

Servings: 4

Ingredients:

2 pounds salad greens, torn

4 cups blueberries

3 cups orange, peeled and cut into segments

2 cups granola

For the vinaigrette:

1 cup blueberries

1 cup olive oil

2 tablespoons coconut sugar

2 teaspoons shallot, minced

½ teaspoon sweet paprika

A pinch of black pepper

Directions:

In your food processor, combine 1 cup blueberries with the oil, sugar, shallot, paprika and black pepper and pulse well. In a salad, bowl, combine 4 cups blueberries with salad greens, granola and oranges and toss.

Add the blueberry vinaigrette, toss and serve for breakfast. Enjoy!

Nutrition: calories 171, fat 2, fiber 4, carbs 8, protein 8

3 Kale Salad with Quinoa

Preparation time: 10 minutes

Cooking time: 0 minutes

Servings: 4

Ingredients:

6 cups kale, chopped

¼ cup lemon juice

½ cup olive oil

1 teaspoon mustard

1 and ½ cups quinoa, cooked

1 and ½ cups cherry tomatoes, halved

A pinch of black pepper

3 tablespoons pine nuts, toasted

Directions:

In a large salad bowl, combine the kale with quinoa and cherry tomatoes.

Add lemon juice, oil, mustard, black pepper and pine nuts, toss well, divide between plates and serve for breakfast. Enjoy!

Nutrition: calories 165, fat 5, fiber 7, carbs 14, protein 6

4 Salmon Breakfast Salad

Preparation time: 10 minutes

Cooking time: 0 minutes

Servings: 2

Ingredients:

3 tablespoons nonfat yogurt

1 teaspoon horseradish sauce

1 tablespoon dill, chopped

1 teaspoon lemon juice

4 ounces smoked salmon, boneless, skinless and torn

3 ounces salad greens

2 ounces cherry tomatoes, halved

2 ounces black olives, pitted and sliced

Directions:

In a salad bowl, combine the salmon with salad greens, tomatoes and black olives.

In another bowl, combine the yogurt with horseradish, dill and lemon juice, whisk well, pour over the salad, toss well and serve for breakfast.

Enjoy!

Nutrition: calories 177, fat 4, fiber 7, carbs 14, protein 8

5 Pear and Banana Salad

Preparation time: 10 minutes

Cooking time: 0 minutes

Servings: 2

Ingredients:

1 banana, peeled and sliced

1 Asian pear, cored and cubed

Juice of ½ lime

½ teaspoon cinnamon powder

2 ounces pepitas, toasted

Directions:

In a bowl, combine the banana with the pear, lime juice, cinnamon and pepitas, toss, divide between small plates and serve for breakfast.

Enjoy!

Nutrition: calories 188, fat 2, fiber 3, carbs 5, protein 7

6 Easy Plum And Avocado Salad

Preparation time: 10 minutes

Cooking time: 0 minutes

Servings: 3

Ingredients:

2 avocados, peeled, pitted and cubed

4 plums, stones removed and cubed

1 cup cilantro, chopped

1 garlic clove, minced

Juice of 1 lemon

A drizzle of olive oil

1 red chili pepper, minced

Directions:

In a salad bowl, combine the avocados with plums, cilantro, garlic, lemon juice, oil and chili pepper, toss well, divide between plates and serve for breakfast.

Enjoy!

Nutrition: calories 212, fat 2, fiber 4, carbs 14, protein 11

7 Quinoa Bowls

Preparation time: 10 minutes

Cooking time: 20 minutes

Servings: 2

Ingredients:

1 peach, sliced

1/3 cup quinoa, rinsed

2/3 cup low-fat milk

½ teaspoon vanilla extract

2 teaspoons brown sugar

12 raspberries

14 blueberries

Directions:

In a small pan, combine the quinoa with the milk, sugar and vanilla, stir, bring to a simmer over medium heat, cover the pan, cook for 20 minutes and flip with a fork.

Divide this mix into 2 bowls, top each with raspberries and blueberries and serve for breakfast.

Enjoy!

Nutrition: calories 177, fat 2, fiber 4, carbs 9, protein 8

Soup

8 Chicken Corn Chowder

Preparation Time: 10 MINUTES

Cooking Time: 8 HOURS

Servings: 6

Ingredients:

1-pound boneless, skinless chicken thighs, cut into 1-inch pieces

2 onions, chopped

3 jalapeño peppers, seeded and minced

2 red bell peppers, seeded and chopped

11/2 cups fresh or frozen corn

6 cups Poultry Broth (here), or store bought

1 teaspoon garlic powder

1/2 teaspoon sea salt

1/4 teaspoons freshly ground black pepper

1 cup skim milk

Directions:

In your slow cooker, combine the chicken, onions, jalapeños, red bell peppers, corn, broth, garlic powder, salt, and pepper.

Cover and cook on low for 8 hours.

Stir in the skim milk just before serving.

Nutrition: Calories: 236; Total Fat: 6g; Saturated Fat: 2g; Cholesterol: 68mg; Carbohydrates: 17g; Fiber: 3g; Protein: 27g

9 Turkey Ginger Soup

Preparation Time: 10 MINUTES

Cooking Time: 8 HOURS

Servings: 6

Ingredients:

1 pound boneless, skinless turkey thighs, cut into 1-inch pieces

1 pound fresh shiitake mushrooms, halved

3 carrots, peeled and sliced

2 cups frozen peas

1 tablespoon grated fresh ginger

6 cups Poultry Broth (here), or store bought

1 tablespoon low-sodium soy sauce

1 teaspoon toasted sesame oil

2 teaspoons garlic powder

11/2 cups cooked Brown Rice (here)

Directions:

In your slow cooker, combine the turkey, mushrooms, carrots, peas, ginger, broth, soy sauce, sesame oil, and garlic powder. Cover and cook on low for 8 hours.

About 30 minutes before serving, stir in the rice to warm it through.

Nutrition: Calories: 318; Total Fat: 7g; Saturated Fat: 0g; Cholesterol: 0mg; Carbohydrates: 42g; Fiber: 6g; Protein: 24g

10   Taco Soup

Preparation Time: 15 minutes

Cooking Time: 8 hours

Servings: 6

Ingredients:

1 pound ground turkey breast

1 onion, chopped

1 (14-ounce) can tomatoes and green chiles, with their juice

6 cups Poultry Broth (here), or store bought

1 teaspoon chili powder

1 teaspoon ground cumin

1/2 teaspoon sea salt

1/4 cup chopped fresh cilantro

Juice of 1 lime

1/2 cup grated low-fat Cheddar cheese

Directions:

Crumble the turkey into the slow cooker.

Add the onion, tomatoes and green chiles (with their juice), broth, chili powder, cumin, and salt.

Cover and cook on low for 8 hours.

Stir in the cilantro and lime juice.

Serve garnished with the cheese.

Nutrition: Calories: 281; Total Fat: 10g; Saturated Fat: 4g; Cholesterol: 66mg; Carbohydrates: 20g; Fiber: 5g; Protein: 30g

11   Italian Sausage & Fennel Soup

Preparation Time: 10 minutes

Cooking Time: 8 hours

Servings: 6

Ingredients:

1-pound Italian chicken or turkey sausage, cut into 1/2-inch slices

2 onions, chopped

1 fennel bulb, chopped

6 cups Poultry Broth (here), or store bought

1/4 cup dry sherry

11/2 teaspoons garlic powder

1 teaspoon dried thyme

1/2 teaspoon sea salt

1/4 teaspoons freshly ground black pepper

Pinch red pepper flakes

Directions:

In your slow cooker, combine all the ingredients.

Cover and cook on low for 8 hours.

Nutrition: Calories: 311; Total Fat: 22g; Saturated Fat: 7g; Cholesterol: 64mg; Carbohydrates: 8g; Fiber: 2g; Protein: 18g

12   Pork, Fennel & Apple Stew

Preparation Time: 15 MINUTES

Cooking Time: 8 HOURS

Servings: 6

Ingredients:

1 pound pork shoulder, trimmed of as much fat as possible and cut into 1-inch cubes

2 sweet-tart apples (such as Braeburn), peeled, cored, and sliced

1 fennel bulb, sliced

2 red onions, sliced

1/4 cup apple cider vinegar

2 cups Poultry Broth (here), or store bought

1 teaspoon garlic powder

1 teaspoon ground mustard

1/2 teaspoon ground cinnamon

1/2 teaspoon sea salt

1/8 teaspoon freshly ground black pepper

Directions:

In your slow cooker, combine all the ingredients.

Cover and cook on low for 8 hours.

Nutrition: Calories: 297; Total Fat: 11g; Saturated Fat: 4g;

Cholesterol: 76mg; Carbohydrates: 15g; Fiber: 4g; Protein: 21g

---

Poultry

13   Southwestern Chicken and Pasta

Preparation time: 10 minutes

Cooking time: 10 minutes

Servings: 2

Ingredients:

1 cup uncooked whole-wheat rigatoni

2 chicken breasts, cut into cubes

1/4 cup of salsa

1 1/2 cups of canned unsalted tomato sauce

1/8 tsp garlic powder

1 tsp cumin

1/2 tsp chili powder

1/2 cup canned black beans, drained

1/2 cup fresh corn

1/4 cup Monterey Jack and Colby cheese, shredded

Directions:

Fill a pot with water up to ¾ full and boil it. Add pasta to cook until it is al dente, then drain the pasta while rinsing under cold water. Preheat a skillet with cooking oil, then cook the chicken for 10 minutes until golden from both sides.

Add tomato sauce, salsa, cumin, garlic powder, black beans, corn, and chili powder. Cook the mixture while stirring, then toss in the pasta. Serve with 2 tablespoons cheese on top. Enjoy.

Nutrition: Calories 245 Fat 16.3 g Sodium 515 mg Carbs 19.3 g Protein 33.3 g

14   Stuffed Chicken Breasts

Preparation time: 15 minutes

Cooking time: 30 minutes

Servings: 4

Ingredients:

3 tbsp seedless raisins

1/2 cup of chopped onion

1/2 cup of chopped celery

1/4 tsp garlic, minced

1 bay leaf

1 cup apple with peel, chopped

2 tbsp chopped water chestnuts

4 large chicken breast halves, 5 ounces each

1 tablespoon olive oil

1 cup fat-free milk

1 teaspoon curry powder

2 tablespoons all-purpose (plain) flour

1 lemon, cut into 4 wedges

Directions:

Set the oven to heat at 425 degrees F. Grease a baking dish with cooking oil. Soak raisins in warm water until they swell. Grease a heated skillet with cooking spray.

Add celery, garlic, onions, and bay leaf. Sauté for 5 minutes. Discard the bay leaf, then toss in apples. Stir cook for 2 minutes. Drain the soaked raisin and pat them dry to remove excess water.

Add raisins and water chestnuts to the apple mixture. Pull apart the chicken's skin and stuff the apple raisin mixture between the skin and the chicken. Preheat olive oil in another skillet and sear the breasts for 5 minutes per side.

Place the chicken breasts in the baking dish and cover the dish. Bake for 15 minutes until temperature reaches 165 degrees F. Prepare sauce by mixing milk, flour, and curry powder in a saucepan.

Stir cook until the mixture thickens, about 5 minutes. Pour this sauce over the baked chicken. Bake again in the covered dish for 10 minutes. Serve.

Nutrition: Calories 357 Fat 32.7 g Sodium 277 mg Carbs 17.7 g Protein 31.2 g

15   Buffalo Chicken Salad Wrap

Preparation time: 10 minutes

Cooking time: 10 minutes

Servings: 4

Ingredients:

3-4 ounces chicken breasts

2 whole chipotle peppers

1/4 cup white wine vinegar

1/4 cup low-calorie mayonnaise

2 stalks celery, diced

2 carrots, cut into matchsticks

1 small yellow onion, diced

1/2 cup thinly sliced rutabaga or another root vegetable

4 ounces spinach, cut into strips

2 whole-grain tortillas (12-inch diameter)

Directions:

Set the oven or a grill to heat at 375 degrees F. Bake the chicken first for 10 minutes per side. Blend chipotle peppers with mayonnaise and wine vinegar in the blender. Dice the baked chicken into cubes or small chunks.

Mix the chipotle mixture with all the ingredients except tortillas and spinach. Spread 2 ounces of spinach over the tortilla and scoop the stuffing on top. Wrap the tortilla and cut it into half. Serve.

Nutrition: Calories 300 Fat 16.4 g Sodium 471 mg Carbs 8.7 g Protein 38.5 g

16   Chicken Sliders

Preparation time: 10 minutes

Cooking time: 10 minutes

Servings: 4

Ingredients:

10 ounces ground chicken breast

1 tablespoon black pepper

1 tablespoon minced garlic

1 tablespoon balsamic vinegar

1/2 cup minced onion

1 fresh chili pepper, minced

1 tablespoon fennel seed, crushed

4 whole-wheat mini buns

4 lettuce leaves

4 tomato slices

Directions:

Combine all the ingredients except the wheat buns, tomato, and lettuce. Mix well and refrigerate the mixture for 1 hour. Divide the mixture into 4 patties.

Broil these patties in a greased baking tray until golden brown. Place the chicken patties in the wheat buns along with lettuce and tomato. Serve.

Nutrition: Calories 224 Fat 4.5 g Sodium 212 mg Carbs 10.2 g Protein 67.4 g

17   White Chicken Chili

Preparation time: 20 minutes

Cooking time: 15 minutes

Servings: 4

Ingredients:

1 can white chunk chicken

2 cans low-sodium white beans, drained

1 can low-sodium diced tomatoes

4 cups of low-sodium chicken broth

1 medium onion, chopped

1/2 medium green pepper, chopped

1 medium red pepper, chopped

2 garlic cloves, minced

2 teaspoons chili powder

1 teaspoon ground cumin

1 teaspoon dried oregano

Cayenne pepper, to taste

8 tablespoons shredded reduced-fat Monterey Jack cheese

3 tablespoons chopped fresh cilantro

Directions:

In a soup pot, add beans, tomatoes, chicken, and chicken broth. Cover this soup pot and let it simmer over medium heat. Meanwhile, grease a nonstick pan with cooking spray. Add peppers, garlic, and onions. Sauté for 5 minutes until soft.

Transfer the mixture to the soup pot. Add cumin, chili powder, cayenne pepper, and oregano. Cook for 10 minutes, then garnish the chili with cilantro and 1 tablespoon cheese. Serve.

Nutrition: Calories 225 Fat 12.9 g Sodium 480 mg Carbs 24.7 g Protein 25.3g

Seafood

18   Scallops and Strawberry Mix

Preparation time: 10 minutes

Cooking time: 6 minutes

Servings: 2

Ingredients:

4 ounces scallops

½ cup Pico de gallo

½ cup strawberries, chopped

1 tablespoon lime juice

Black pepper to the taste

Directions:

Heat up a pan over medium heat, add scallops, cook for 3 minutes on each side and take off heat,

In a bowl, mix strawberries with lime juice, Pico de gallo, scallops and pepper, toss and serve cold.

Enjoy!

Nutrition: calories 169, fat 2, fiber 2, carbs 8, protein 13

19   Baked Haddock with Avocado Mayonnaise

Preparation time: 10 minutes

Cooking time: 30 minutes

Servings: 4

Ingredients:

1 pound haddock, boneless

3 teaspoons water

2 tablespoons lemon juice

A pinch of salt and black pepper

2 tablespoons avocado mayonnaise

1 teaspoon dill, chopped

Cooking spray

Directions:

Spray a baking dish with some cooking oil, add fish, water, lemon juice, salt, black pepper, mayo and dill, toss, introduce in the oven and bake at 350 degrees F for 30 minutes.

Divide between plates and serve.

Enjoy!

Nutrition: calories 264, fat 4, fiber 5, carbs 7, protein 12

20   Basil Tilapia

Preparation time: 10 minutes

Cooking time: 10 minutes

Servings: 4

Ingredients:

4 tilapia fillets, boneless

Black pepper to the taste

½ cup low-fat parmesan, grated

4 tablespoons avocado mayonnaise

2 teaspoons basil, dried

2 tablespoons lemon juice

¼ cup olive oil

Directions:

Grease a baking dish with the oil, add tilapia fillets, black pepper, spread mayo, basil, drizzle lemon juice and top with the parmesan, introduce in preheated broiler and cook over medium-high heat for 5 minutes on each side.

Divide between plates and serve with a side salad.

Enjoy!

Nutrition: calories 215, fat 10, fiber 5, carbs 7, protein 11

21   Salmon Meatballs with Garlic

Preparation time: 10 minutes

Cooking time: 30 minutes

Servings: 4

Ingredients:

Cooking spray

2 garlic cloves, minced

1 yellow onion, chopped

1 pound wild salmon, boneless and minced

¼ cup chives, chopped

1 egg

2 tablespoons Dijon mustard

1 tablespoon coconut flour

A pinch of salt and black pepper

Directions:

In a bowl, mix onion with garlic, salmon, chives, coconut flour, salt, pepper, mustard and egg, stir well, shape medium meatballs, arrange them on a baking sheet, grease them with cooking spray, introduce in the oven at 350 degrees F and bake for 25 minutes.

Divide the meatballs between plates and serve with a side salad.

Enjoy!

Nutrition: calories 211, fat 4, fiber 1, carbs 6, protein 13

22   Mushroom Florentine

Preparation time: 15 minutes

Cooking time: 20 minutes

Servings: 4

Ingredients:

5 oz whole-grain pasta

¼ cup low-sodium vegetable broth

1 cup mushrooms, sliced

¼ cup of soy milk

1 teaspoon olive oil

½ teaspoon Italian seasonings

Directions:

1. Cook the pasta according to the direction of the manufacturer. Then pour olive oil into the saucepan and heat it. Add mushrooms and Italian seasonings. Stir the mushrooms well and cook for 10 minutes.

 2. Then add soy milk and vegetable broth. Add cooked pasta and mix up the mixture well. Cook it for 5 minutes on low heat.

Nutrition: Calories 287 Protein 12.4g Carbohydrates 50.4g Fat 4.2g Sodium 26mg

23   Hasselback Eggplant

Preparation time: 15 minutes

Cooking time: 25 minutes

Servings: 2

Ingredients:

2 eggplants, trimmed

2 tomatoes, sliced

1 tablespoon low-fat yogurt

1 teaspoon curry powder

1 teaspoon olive oil

Directions:

1. Make the cuts in the eggplants in the shape of the Hasselback. Then rub the vegetables with curry powder and fill with sliced tomatoes. Sprinkle the eggplants with olive oil and yogurt and wrap in the foil (each Hasselback eggplant wrap separately). Bake the vegetables at 375F for 25 minutes. Nutrition: Calories 188 Protein 7g Carbohydrates 38.1g Fat 3g Sodium 23mg

24   Vegetarian Kebabs

Preparation time: 15 minutes

Cooking time: 6 minutes

Servings: 4

Ingredients:

2 tablespoons balsamic vinegar

1 tablespoon olive oil

1 teaspoon dried parsley

2 tablespoons water

2 sweet peppers

2 red onions, peeled

2 zucchinis, trimmed

Directions:

1. Cut the sweet peppers and onions into medium size squares. Then slice the zucchini. String all vegetables into the skewers. After this, in the shallow bowl, mix up olive oil, dried parsley, water, and balsamic vinegar.

 2. Sprinkle the vegetable skewers with olive oil mixture and transfer in the preheated to 390F grill. Cook the kebabs within 3 minutes per side or until the vegetables are light brown.

Nutrition: Calories 88 Protein 2.4g Carbohydrates 13g Fat 3.9g Sodium 14mg

25   White Beans Stew

Preparation time: 15 minutes

Cooking time: 55 minutes

Servings: 4

Ingredients:

1 cup white beans, soaked

1 cup low-sodium vegetable broth

1 cup zucchini, chopped

1 teaspoon tomato paste

1 tablespoon avocado oil

4 cups of water

½ teaspoon peppercorns

½ teaspoon ground black pepper

¼ teaspoon ground nutmeg

Directions:

1. Heat avocado oil in the saucepan, add zucchinis, and roast them for 5 minutes. After this, add white beans, vegetable broth, tomato paste, water, peppercorns, ground black pepper, and ground nutmeg. Simmer the stew within 50 minutes on low heat.

Nutrition: Calories 184 Protein 12.3g Carbohydrates 32.6g Fat 1g Sodium 55mg

26   Vegetarian Lasagna

Preparation time: 15 minutes

Cooking time: 30 minutes

Servings: 6

Ingredients:

1 cup carrot, diced

½ cup bell pepper, diced

1 cup spinach, chopped

1 tablespoon olive oil

1 teaspoon chili powder

1 cup tomatoes, chopped

4 oz low-fat cottage cheese

1 eggplant, sliced

1 cup low-sodium vegetable broth

Directions:

1. Put carrot, bell pepper, and spinach in the saucepan. Add olive oil and chili powder and stir the vegetables well. Cook them for 5 minutes.

2. Make the sliced eggplant layer in the casserole mold and top it with vegetable mixture. Add tomatoes, vegetable stock, and cottage cheese. Bake the lasagna for 30 minutes at 375F.

Nutrition: Calories 77 Protein 4.1g Carbohydrates 9.7g Fat 3g Sodium 124mg

27   Carrot Cakes

Preparation time: 15 minutes

Cooking time: 10 minutes

Servings: 4

Ingredients:

1 cup carrot, grated

1 tablespoon semolina

1 egg, beaten

1 teaspoon Italian seasonings

1 tablespoon sesame oil

Directions:

1. In the mixing bowl, mix up grated carrot, semolina, egg, and Italian seasonings. Heat sesame oil in the skillet. Make the carrot cakes with the help of 2 spoons and put in the skillet. Roast the cakes for 4 minutes per side.

Nutrition: Calories 70 Protein 1.9g Carbohydrates 4.8g Fat 4.9g Sodium 35mg

---

Side Dishes, Salads & Appetizers

28   Mashed Potatoes

Preparation time: 10 minutes

Cooking time: 20 minutes

Servings: 6

Ingredients:

3 pounds potatoes, peeled and cubed

2 tablespoons non-fat butter

½ cup coconut milk

A pinch of salt and black pepper

½ cup low-fat sour cream

Directions:

Put the potatoes in a pot, add water to cover, add a pinch of salt and pepper, bring to a boil over medium heat, cook for 20 minutes and drain.

Add butter, milk and sour cream, mash well, stir everything, divide between plates and serve as a side dish.

Enjoy!

Nutrition: calories 188, fat 3, fiber 7, carbs 14, protein 8

29 Squash Salad with Orange

Preparation time: 10 minutes

Cooking time: 30 minutes

Servings: 6

Ingredients:

1 cup orange juice

3 tablespoons coconut sugar

1 and ½ tablespoons mustard

1 tablespoon ginger, grated

1 and ½ pounds butternut squash, peeled and roughly cubed

Cooking spray

A pinch of black pepper

1/3 cup olive oil

6 cups salad greens

1 radicchio, sliced

½ cup pistachios, roasted

Directions:

In a bowl, combine the orange juice with the sugar, mustard, ginger, black pepper and squash, toss well, spread on a lined baking sheet, spray everything with cooking oil, introduce in the oven and bake at 400 degrees F for 30 minutes.

In a salad bowl, combine the squash with salad greens, radicchio, pistachios and oil, toss well, divide between plates and serve as a side dish.

Enjoy!

Nutrition: calories 275, fat 3, fiber 4, carbs 16, protein 6

30   Colored Iceberg Salad

Preparation time: 10 minutes

Cooking time: 0 minutes

Servings: 4

Ingredients:

1 iceberg lettuce head, leaves torn

6 bacon slices, cooked and halved

2 green onions, sliced

3 carrots, shredded

6 radishes, sliced

¼ cup red vinegar

¼ cup olive oil

3 garlic cloves, minced

A pinch of black pepper

Directions:

In a large salad bowl, combine the lettuce leaves with the bacon, green onions, carrots, radishes, vinegar, oil, garlic and black pepper, toss, divide between plates and serve as a side dish.

Enjoy!

Nutrition: calories 235, fat 4, fiber 4, carbs 10, protein 6

31   Fennel Salad with Arugula

Preparation time: 10 minutes

Cooking time: 0 minutes

Servings: 4

Ingredients:

2 fennel bulbs, trimmed and shaved

1 and ¼ cups zucchini, sliced

2/3 cup dill, chopped

¼ cup lemon juice

¼ cup olive oil

6 cups arugula

½ cups walnuts, chopped

1/3 cup low-fat feta cheese, crumbled

Directions:

In a large bowl, combine the fennel with the zucchini, dill, lemon juice, arugula, oil, walnuts and cheese, toss, divide between plates and serve as a side dish.

Enjoy!

Nutrition: calories 188, fat 4, fiber 5, carbs 14, protein 6

32   Corn Mix

Preparation time: 10 minutes

Cooking time: 0 minutes

Servings: 4

Ingredients:

½ cup cider vinegar

¼ cup coconut sugar

A pinch of black pepper

4 cups corn

½ cup red onion, chopped

½ cup cucumber, sliced

½ cup red bell pepper, chopped

½ cup cherry tomatoes, halved

3 tablespoons parsley, chopped

1 tablespoon basil, chopped

1 tablespoon jalapeno, chopped

2 cups baby arugula leaves

Directions:

In a large bowl, combine the corn with onion, cucumber, bell pepper, cherry tomatoes, parsley, basil, jalapeno and arugula and toss.

Add vinegar, sugar and black pepper, toss well, divide between plates and serve as a side dish.

Enjoy!

Nutrition: calories 100, fat 2, fiber 3, carbs 14, protein 4

33   Persimmon Salad

Preparation time: 10 minutes

Cooking time: 0 minutes

Servings: 4

Ingredients:

Seeds from 1 pomegranate

2 persimmons, cored and sliced

5 cups baby arugula

6 tablespoons green onions, chopped

4 navel oranges, peeled and cut into segments

¼ cup white vinegar

1/3 cup olive oil

3 tablespoons pine nuts

1 and ½ teaspoons orange zest, grated

2 tablespoons orange juice

1 tablespoon coconut sugar

½ shallot, chopped

A pinch of cinnamon powder

Directions:

In a salad bowl, combine the pomegranate seeds with persimmons, arugula, green onions and oranges and toss.

In another bowl, combine the vinegar with the oil, pine nuts, orange zest, orange juice, sugar, shallot and cinnamon, whisk well, add to the salad, toss and serve as a side dish.

Enjoy!

Nutrition: calories 188, fat 4, fiber 4, carbs 14, protein 4

34   Avocado Side Salad

Preparation time: 10 minutes

Cooking time: 0 minutes

Servings: 4

Ingredients:

4 blood oranges, peeled and cut into segments

2 tablespoons olive oil

A pinch of red pepper, crushed

2 avocados, peeled, pitted and cut into wedges

1 and ½ cups baby arugula

¼ cup almonds, toasted and chopped

1 tablespoon lemon juice

Directions:

In a bowl, combine the oranges with the oil, red pepper, avocados, arugula, almonds and lemon juice, toss, divide between plates and serve as a side dish.

Enjoy!

Nutrition: calories 231, fat 4, fiber 8, carbs 16, protein 6

35   Corn and Beans Salad

Preparation time: 10 minutes

Cooking time: 0 minutes

Servings: 4

Ingredients:

3 garlic cloves, minced

Juice of ½ lemon

6 ounces coconut cream

2 lettuce hearts, torn

1 cup corn

4 ounces green beans, halved

1 cup cherry tomatoes, halved

1 cucumber, chopped

1/3 cup chives, chopped

1 avocado, peeled, pitted and halved

6 bacon slices, cooked and chopped

Directions:

In a bowl, combine the lettuce with corn, green beans, cherry tomatoes, cucumber, chives, avocado and bacon and toss.

In another bowl, combine the garlic with lemon juice and coconut cream, whisk well, add to the salad, toss and serve as a side dish.

Enjoy!

Nutrition: calories 175, fat 12, fiber 4, carbs 13, protein 6

36   Easy Kale Mix

Preparation time: 10 minutes

Cooking time: 0 minutes

Servings: 4

Ingredients:

1 whole wheat bread slice, toasted and torn into small pieces

6 tablespoons low-fat cheddar, grated

3 tablespoons olive oil

5 tablespoons lemon juice

1 garlic clove, minced

7 cups kale, torn

A pinch of black pepper

Directions:

In a bowl, combine the bread with cheese and kale.

In another bowl, combine the oil with the lemon juice, garlic and black pepper, whisk, add to the salad, toss, divide between plates and serve as a side dish.

Enjoy!

Nutrition: calories 200, fat 4, fiber 5, carbs 14, protein 8

37   Asparagus with Edamame Salad

Preparation time: 10 minutes

Cooking time: 4 minutes

Servings: 4

Ingredients:

4 tablespoons avocado oil

2 tablespoons balsamic vinegar

1 tablespoon coconut aminos

1 garlic clove, minced

1 pound asparagus, trimmed

6 cups frisee lettuce leaves, torn

1 cup edamame, shelled

1 cup parsley, chopped

Directions:

Heat up a pan with 1 tablespoon oil over medium-high heat, add asparagus, cook for 4 minutes and transfer to a salad bowl.

Add lettuce, edammae and parsley and toss.

In another bowl, combine the rest of the oil with the vinegar, aminos and garlic, whisk well, add over the salad, toss, divide between plates and serve as a side dish.

Enjoy!

Nutrition: calories 200, fat 4, fiber 5, carbs 14, protein 6

Dessert and Snacks

38   Jalapeno Crisp For Keto Goers

Preparation time: 10 minutes

Cooking Time: 1 hour 15 minutes

Serving: 20

Ingredients:

1 cup sesame seeds

1 cup sunflower seeds

1 cup flaxseeds

½ cup hulled hemp seeds

3 tablespoons Psyllium husk

1 teaspoon salt

1 teaspoon baking powder

2 cups water

Directions:

Preheat your oven to 350 degrees F.

Take your blender and add seeds, baking powder, salt and Psyllium husk.

Blend well until a sand-like texture appears.

Stir in water and mix until a batter forms.

Allow the batter to rest for 10 minutes until a dough like thick mixture forms.

Pour the dough onto cookie sheet lined up with parchment paper.

Spread evenly, making sure that it has a ¼ inch thickness all around.

Bake for 75 minutes in the oven.

Remove and cut into 20 spices.

Allow them to cool for 30 minutes and enjoy!

Nutrition:

Calories: 156

Fat: 13g

Carbohydrates: 2g

Protein: 5g

39   Spicy Chicken Fingers

Preparation time: 20 minutes

Cooking Time: 30 minutes

Serving: 4

Ingredients:

1 ¼ pounds, skinless boneless chicken breast tenders

¼ teaspoon salt 1/8 teaspoon fresh ground black pepper

3 cups brown rice cereal

½ cup honey

2 teaspoons sriracha

Directions:

Preheat your oven to 375 degrees F.

Take a baking sheet and coat with cooking spray.

Sprinkle both sides of chicken with salt and pepper.

Transfer brown rice cereal in a re-sealable bag and use rolling pin to crush cereal into pieces.

Pour crushed cereal into a large bowl.

Take a medium bowl and whisk in honey and sriracha.

Dip chicken tenders in honey mix, then dredge in cereal mix.

Place tenders on baking sheet, leaving about ½ inch gap between each tender.

Bake for 30 minutes until the internal temperature reaches 165 degrees F.

Serve and enjoy!

Nutrition:

Calories: 331

Fat: 4g

Carbohydrates: 41g

Protein: 33g

40   Lovely Carrot Cake

Preparation time: 3 hours 15 minutes

Cooking Time: Nil

Serving: 6

Ingredients: For Cashew Frosting

2 tablespoons lemon juice

2 cups cashews, soaked

2 tablespoons coconut oil, melted

1/3 cup maple syrup

water

For Cake

1 cup pineapple, dried and chopped

2 carrots, chopped

1 ½ cups coconut flour

1 cup dates, pitted

½ cup dry coconut

½ teaspoon cinnamon

Directions:

Add cashews, lemon juice, maple syrup, coconut oil, apple and pulse well.

Transfer to a bowl and keep it on the side.

Add carrots to your processor and pulse a few times.

Add flour, dates, pineapple, coconut, cinnamon and pulse.

Pour half of the mixture into a spring form pan and spread well.

Add 1/3 of the cashew frosting and spread evenly.

Add remaining cake batter and spread the frosting.

Place in your freezer until it is hard.

Cut and serve.

Enjoy!

Nutrition:

Calories: 140

Fat: 4g

Carbohydrates: 8g

Protein: 4g

41   Grilled Peach with Honey Yogurt

Dressing

Preparation time: 10 minutes

Cooking Time: 5 minutes

Serving: 6

Ingredients:

2 large peaches, ripe and halved

2 tablespoons honey

1/8 teaspoon cinnamon

¼ cut vanilla Greek yogurt, fat free

Directions:

Prepare your outdoor grill and heat on low heat.

Grill your peaches on indirect heat until they are t

should take about 2-4 minutes each side.

Take a bowl and mix in yogurt and cinnamon

Drizzle honey mix on top and enjoy!

Nutrition:

Calories: 140

Fat: 4g

Carbohydrates: 8g

Protein: 4g

Preparation time: 10 minutes

Cooking Time: 15 minutes

Serving: 6

Ingredients:

½ cup packed light brown sugar

½ cup sugar

½ cup oil

½ cup apple sauce

2 whole eggs

cup flour

teaspoon vanilla

teaspoon baking soda

whole wheat flour

poon salt

oon ground nutmeg

on cinnamon, ground

carrots, grated

en raisin

d oats, raw

oven to about 350 degrees F.

d mix in applesauce, oil, sugar, vanilla and

Take another bowl and mix in the dry ingredients.

Blend the dry ingredients into the bowl with wet mixture.

Stir in carrots and raisins to the mix.

Take a greased cookie sheet and drop in the mixture spoon by spoon.

Transfer to oven and bake for 15 minutes until you have a golden-brown texture.

Serve and enjoy!

Nutrition:

Calories: 140

Fat: 4g

Carbohydrates: 8g

Protein: 4g

43   Milky Pudding

Preparation time: 10 minutes

Cooking Time: 5-10 minutes + chill time

Serving: 6

Ingredients:

3 tablespoons cornstarch

½ teaspoon vanilla

1/3 cup chocolate chips

2 cups non-fat milk

1/8 teaspoon salt

2 tablespoons salt

2 tablespoons sugar

Directions:

Take a medium sized bowl and add cocoa powder, cornstarch, salt, sugar and mix well.

Whisk in the milk.

Place over medium heat and keep heating until thick and bubbly.

Remove the mixture from heat and stir in vanilla and chocolate chips.

Keep mixing until the chips are melted and you have a smooth pudding.

Pour into a large sized dish and let it chill.

Serve and enjoy!

Nutrition:

Calories: 140

Fat: 4g

Carbohydrates: 8g

Protein: 4g

44 Fresh Honey Strawberries with Yogurt

Preparation time: 10 minutes

Cooking Time: 5-10 minutes + chill time

Serving: 6

Ingredients:

4 tablespoons almond, sliced and toasted

3 cups yogurt, low fat

4 teaspoons honey

1 pint fresh strawberries

Directions:

Take your strawberries and wash under water, clean well.

Cut into quarters.

Take your serving dishes and add ¾ cup yogurt into each dish.

Divide strawberries among the dishes.

Top each dish with honey, sliced almonds.

Serve and enjoy!

Nutrition:

Calories: 140

Fat: 4g

Carbohydrates: 8g

Protein: 4g

45   Hoisin Meatballs

Preparation time: 20 minutes

Cooking Time: 10 minutes

Servings: 2 dozen

Ingredients:

1 cup dry red wine or beef broth of choice

2 tablespoons soy sauce

4 chopped green onions

¼ cup minced cilantro

¼ cup chopped onion

1 lightly beaten egg

3 tablespoons hoisin sauce

2 minced garlic cloves

½ teaspoon salt and pepper each

1 pound ground beef

1 pound ground pork of choice

sesame seeds for topping

Directions:

In instant pot, put the wine, sauces, and boil them, then reduce heat.

Combine next 7 ingredients in bowl, then mix it together with the meats, shaping into meatballs, and then put it in instant pot.

Set it to manual high pressure for 10 minutes, quick release, and then top with sesame seeds.

Nutrition: Calories: 78, Fat: 5g, Carbs: 1g, Net Carbs: 1g, Protein: 6g, Fiber: 0g

46   Cuban Pulled Pork Sandwiches:

Preparation time: 20 minutes

Cooking Time: 25 minutes

Servings: 16

Ingredients:

3 cups yogurt, low fat

4 teaspoons honey

1 pint fresh strawberries

Directions:

Take your strawberries and wash under water, clean well. Cut into quarters.

Take your serving dishes and add ¾ cup yogurt into each dish.

Divide strawberries among the dishes.

Top each dish with honey, sliced almonds.

Serve and enjoy!

Nutrition:

Calories: 140

Fat: 4g

Carbohydrates: 8g

Protein: 4g

45   Hoisin Meatballs

Preparation time: 20 minutes

Cooking Time: 10 minutes

Servings: 2 dozen

Ingredients:

1 cup dry red wine or beef broth of choice

2 tablespoons soy sauce

4 chopped green onions

¼ cup minced cilantro

¼ cup chopped onion

1 lightly beaten egg

3 tablespoons hoisin sauce

2 minced garlic cloves

½ teaspoon salt and pepper each

1 pound ground beef

1 pound ground pork of choice

sesame seeds for topping

Directions:

In instant pot, put the wine, sauces, and boil them, then reduce heat.

Combine next 7 ingredients in bowl, then mix it together with the meats, shaping into meatballs, and then put it in instant pot.

Set it to manual high pressure for 10 minutes, quick release, and then top with sesame seeds.

Nutrition: Calories: 78, Fat: 5g, Carbs: 1g, Net Carbs: 1g, Protein: 6g, Fiber: 0g

46 Cuban Pulled Pork Sandwiches:

Preparation time: 20 minutes

Cooking Time: 25 minutes

Servings: 16

Ingredients:

1 boneless pork shoulder butt roast

2 teaspoons salt and pepper

1 cup orange juice

½ cup lime juice

1 tablespoon olive oil

12 minced garlic cloves

2 tablespoons ground coriander

1 teaspoon cayenne pepper

2 teaspoons white pepper

for the sandwiches:

2 loaves French bread

16 dill pickle slices

1 pound sliced Swiss cheese

1 pound sliced deli ham

Mustard for topping

Directions:

Cut pork into small, 2-inch pieces, and season with salt and pepper, then brown it in the instant pot after turning it onto sauté.

Add in the juices, and scrape the brown bits, then add the garlic, coriander, white pepper, and the cayenne pepper, and then put pork in there, and then cook it on manual high pressure for 25 minutes.

When finished, do a natural pressure release, and then quick release it, and then shred with forks, and then remove a cup of the liquid, and then toss this together.

Prepare sandwiches with the bread halves, then pickles, ham, pork, cheese, and then the tops.

Nutrition: Calories: 573, Fat: 28g, Carbs: 35g, Net Carbs: 33g, Protein: 45g, Fiber: 2g

47　　Cinnamon Baked Apples with Walnuts

Preparation time: 10 minutes

Cooking time: 25 minutes

Servings: 4

Ingredients:

4 firm apples, such as Cortland or Granny Smith, peeled and cored

3 teaspoons light brown sugar

½ teaspoon cinnamon

½ teaspoon cardamom

1 cup unsweetened apple cider

1 cup unsweetened orange juice

1 tablespoon cornstarch

2 tablespoons cold water

2 tablespoons chopped black walnuts

Direction

Preheat oven to 350°F (180°C).

Place apples in a lined baking pan, and sprinkle with brown sugar, cinnamon, and cardamom.

Pour cider and orange juice into the dish and bake for 20 to 25 minutes. Remove apples to 4 dessert dishes and set aside.

Pour baking juices into a small saucepan, and heat on medium heat to a low simmer. In a separate bowl, mix cornstarch and water, then whisk into pan. Continue stirring until thickened, then spoon over each apple. Sprinkle chopped walnuts over each portion and serve warm.

Nutrition 211 calories 3g fat 2g protein 45g carbs 6mg sodium 21mg potassium

48   Raspberry Walnut Sorbet

Preparation time: 5 minutes

Cooking time: 0 minutes

Servings: 4

Ingredients:

2 cups fresh ripe raspberries

¼ cup chopped walnuts

1 teaspoon lemon juice

2 tablespoons organic agave nectar

Direction

In a food processor or blender, purée all ingredients together.

Freeze in an ice cream maker. Alternately, spread fruit mixture onto a cookie sheet and place in freezer.

Every 20 minutes scrape through fruit mixture with a spoon so that it doesn't freeze into a solid mass (this will keep it nice and light).

Nutrition 75 calories 4g fat 2g protein 9g carbohydrates 1mg sodium 18mg potassium

49   Vanilla Pumpkin Pudding

Preparation time: 5 minutes

Cooking time: 0 minutes

Servings: 6

Ingredients:

1½ cups fat-free vanilla yogurt

1 (20-ounce / 567-g) can plain pumpkin purée

½ teaspoon ground nutmeg

½ teaspoon ground cinnamon

1 vanilla bean

Direction

Combine yogurt, pumpkin purée, nutmeg, and cinnamon in a medium-sized mixing bowl. Scrape vanilla beans out of husk and into mixture. Mix well until all ingredients are combined. Chill until ready to serve.

Nutrition 95 calories 1.1g fat 4.1g protein 17g carbohydrates 38mg sodium 61mg potassium

Preparation time: 5 minutes

Cooking time: 12 minutes

Servings: 12

Ingredients:

3 medium egg whites

½ teaspoon cream of tartar

½ cup sugar

½ teaspoon orange extract

1½ tablespoons cocoa powder

6 ounces (170 g) bittersweet chocolate, melted but not hot

Olive oil cooking spray

Direction

Preheat oven to 350°F (180°C).

In a dry, medium-sized glass bowl, beat egg whites and cream of tartar with a hand mixer on medium speed until peaks begin to form, about 1 minute. Add sugar slowly while you continue to mix.

Add orange extract and continue beating, scraping sides of bowl frequently, until mixture forms firm peaks and is glossy. In a separate bowl, stir cocoa into melted chocolate, then gently fold mixture into meringue. Line baking sheets with parchment paper, then apply olive oil cooking spray. Drop rounded spoonsful of mixture onto parchment paper.

Bake on middle rack for 8 to 12 minutes until puffs are firm on outside but still soft on inside. You may want to switch to the top rack for the last couple of minutes so that the bottoms don't brown. When puffs are cool, remove from parchment paper, and store in an airtight container for up to 1 week. Nutrition 102 calories 5g fat 2g protein 13g carbohydrates 9mg sodium 16mg potassium

Conclusion

Everything you eat will affect your brain's way of functioning because food gives your body the raw materials to create, rebuild, repair, and function efficiently. For example, oatmeal is highly recommended both for the health of your heart and brain. Oatmeal also contains ferulic acid, a germ and grain bran antioxidant. Ferulic acid seems to be a general protector of the brain cells, and eliminating toxins keeps them supple and responsible. I suppose we'll see more research on this antioxidant.
However, too much fat is not good in your diet, particularly the saturated fats found in whole milk and cream and animal products. Trans fats can be prevented from being found usually in processed foods and margarine and can block blood vessels and reduce circulation. In general, refined foods, processed foods, and junk foods won't help your brain. They often contain excessive salt, contain incorrect fat types, and contain sugar and preservatives. They lack a great deal of nutritional value, including healthy fiber, antioxidants, and essential nutrients.

Now you have everything you need to start a heart healthy DASH diet so that you can live a heart healthy life. There's no reason to worry about or suffer with your condition when there are easy, tasty recipes that can help you to manage them. There's a little something for everyone in this DASH diet cookbook, and the recipes included are sure to delight family and friends alike. Go from comfort foods to something adventurous. After all, if you aren't bored, you're more likely to stick to a diet and make the changes you want to see. There is also too much sugar to be avoided. Too much sugar and fatty sweets may cause metabolic and diabetes syndrome. Both conditions are linked to a higher risk of high blood pressure, cardiovascular diseases, and cognitive problems. You can do nothing for genetic factors that can raise the risk of heart attacks but reduce the risk of creating issues for your brain by maintaining a healthier lifestyle and eating well-nourished.